DIABETES MEAL PLAN FOR THE NEWLY DIAGNOSED

Essential Nutrients and Healthy Options for Diabetes Management: Stress-Free Strategies for Blood Sugar, Weight Loss, and Exercise

Thelma Howard

Table of Contents

Introduction

Understanding Diabetes

The medical condition known as diabetes mellitus, or simply diabetes, is a long-term metabolic disease marked by increased blood sugar levels. It happens when the body is unable to use the insulin it does make, or when it does not produce enough of it. Insulin is a hormone produced by the pancreas that regulates blood sugar (glucose) levels and allows cells to utilize glucose for energy. Understanding the complexities of diabetes is crucial for effective management and prevention of complications.

Types of Diabetes:

1. Type 1 Diabetes: Type 1 diabetes, previously known as juvenile diabetes or insulin-dependent diabetes, typically develops during childhood or adolescence. It occurs when the immune system mistakenly attacks and destroys the insulin-producing beta cells in the pancreas. High blood sugar levels occur from the body producing little to no insulin as a result. Individuals with type 1 diabetes require lifelong insulin therapy for survival.

2. Type 2 Diabetes: Type 2 diabetes, the most common form of diabetes, usually develops in

adulthood, although it is increasingly diagnosed in children and adolescents. In those with type 2 diabetes, the pancreas may not produce enough insulin to counteract the body's resistance to the drug's effects. This results in elevated blood sugar levels. While genetics play a role in type 2 diabetes, lifestyle factors such as obesity, physical inactivity, and poor diet significantly contribute to its development.

3.   Gestational Diabetes: Pregnancy-related hormonal changes and increased insulin resistance raise blood sugar levels, which can result in gestational diabetes. While gestational diabetes usually resolves after childbirth, women who develop it are at higher risk of developing type 2 diabetes later in life. Proper management of gestational diabetes is essential to reduce the risk of complications for both the mother and the baby.

Risk Factors for Diabetes

The following risk factors raise the chance of having diabetes:

Family History: Individuals with a family history of diabetes are at higher risk of developing the condition themselves. Genetics can influence insulin production, insulin resistance, and overall susceptibility to diabetes.

Obesity: Excess body weight, particularly abdominal fat, increases insulin resistance and the risk of developing type 2 diabetes. Maintaining a healthy weight through diet and exercise is crucial for diabetes prevention and management.

Sedentary Lifestyle: Lack of physical activity contributes to obesity and insulin resistance, increasing the risk of type 2 diabetes. Regular exercise improves insulin sensitivity and helps control blood sugar levels.

Unhealthy Diet: Consuming a diet high in processed foods, sugary beverages, and refined carbohydrates can lead to weight gain and insulin resistance. A diet rich in fruits, vegetables, whole grains, lean proteins, and healthy fats is essential for diabetes prevention and management.

Age: Type 2 diabetes is more common as people age, especially beyond the age of 45. Aging is associated with decreased physical activity, muscle mass, and metabolic rate, contributing to insulin resistance and glucose intolerance.

Ethnicity: Certain ethnic groups, including African Americans, Hispanics, Native Americans, and Asian Americans, have a higher prevalence of diabetes compared to Caucasians. Genetic predisposition, cultural factors, and socioeconomic disparities contribute to these differences.

Symptoms of Diabetes

The type and severity of diabetes might affect the symptoms that a person experiences.
 Common symptoms include:

Frequent Urination: Excess glucose in the blood pulls water from the tissues, leading to increased urination (polyuria).

Excessive Thirst: Dehydration resulting from frequent urination can cause excessive thirst (polydipsia).

Increased Hunger: Despite eating, individuals with diabetes may experience persistent hunger (polyphagia) due to the inability of cells to utilize glucose for energy.

Unexplained Weight Loss: In type 1 diabetes, the body breaks down muscle and fat for energy when it cannot use glucose effectively, resulting in unexplained weight loss.

Fatigue: Insufficient energy production from glucose metabolism can cause fatigue and weakness.

Blurred Vision: High blood sugar levels can cause changes in the shape of the lens in the eye, leading to blurred vision.

Slow Wound Healing: Diabetes impairs the body's ability to heal wounds and infections, increasing the risk of complications.

Frequent Infections: High blood sugar levels weaken the immune system, making individuals with diabetes more susceptible to infections, particularly urinary tract infections and yeast infections.

Diagnosis and Screening

Blood tests measuring oral glucose tolerance, glycated hemoglobin (HbA1c) levels, or fasting blood sugar levels are used to diagnose diabetes. Screening for diabetes is recommended for individuals with risk factors such as obesity, family history of diabetes, sedentary lifestyle, and certain ethnic backgrounds. Early detection and diagnosis allow for timely intervention and management to prevent complications.

Complications of Diabetes

Untreated or poorly managed diabetes can lead to various complications affecting multiple organ systems:

Cardiovascular Complications: Diabetes increases the risk of heart disease, stroke, and peripheral artery disease due to damage to blood vessels and elevated cholesterol levels.

Neuropathy: Diabetes can cause nerve damage (neuropathy) resulting in pain, numbness, tingling, and loss of sensation, particularly in the hands and feet.

Nephropathy: Chronic high blood sugar levels can damage the kidneys (nephropathy), leading to kidney failure and the need for dialysis or transplantation.

Retinopathy: Diabetes affects the blood vessels in the retina, leading to diabetic retinopathy, a leading cause of blindness in adults.

Foot Complications: Nerve damage and poor circulation in the feet increase the risk of foot ulcers, infections, and ultimately, amputation.

Skin Conditions: Diabetes increases the risk of various skin conditions, including bacterial and fungal infections, itching, and slow wound healing.

Mental Health: Diabetes is associated with an increased risk of depression, anxiety, and diabetes distress, which can affect quality of life and adherence to treatment.

Management of Diabetes

Effective management of diabetes requires a multidisciplinary approach involving lifestyle modifications, medication, monitoring, and regular medical care:

Healthy Diet: A balanced diet rich in fruits, vegetables, whole grains, lean proteins, and healthy fats helps control blood sugar levels, manage weight, and reduce the risk of complications.

Regular Exercise: Physical activity improves insulin sensitivity, lowers blood sugar levels, reduces cardiovascular risk, and promotes overall well-being.

Medication: Depending on the type and severity of diabetes, medication may be prescribed to lower blood sugar levels, improve insulin sensitivity, or manage complications.

Blood Sugar Monitoring: Regular monitoring of blood sugar levels helps individuals with diabetes understand how their diet, exercise, medication, and stress levels affect their blood sugar levels.

Education and Support: Diabetes self-management education programs provide individuals with the knowledge, skills, and support needed to effectively manage their condition and prevent complications.

Medical Care: Regular medical check-ups, including screenings for complications such as eye exams, kidney function tests, and foot exams, are essential for early detection and management of diabetes-related complications.

In conclusion, diabetes is a complex metabolic disorder characterized by elevated blood sugar levels resulting from insulin deficiency or resistance. Understanding the types, risk factors, symptoms, diagnosis, complications, and management of diabetes is essential for effective prevention, early detection, and optimal management. By adopting a healthy lifestyle, monitoring blood sugar levels

Chapter One

Getting Started with Meal Planning for Diabetes Meal Plan for Newly Diagnosed

Meal planning is a fundamental aspect of diabetes management, especially for individuals who have been newly diagnosed with the condition. Proper meal planning can help regulate blood sugar levels, manage weight, and reduce the risk of complications associated with diabetes. In this comprehensive guide, we will delve into the essential aspects of getting started with meal planning for individuals newly diagnosed with diabetes.

Understanding the Importance of Meal Planning:

Meal planning is the process of organizing and preparing meals in advance to ensure they meet nutritional needs while aligning with dietary goals and preferences. For individuals with diabetes, meal planning plays a crucial role in controlling blood sugar levels by managing carbohydrate intake, portion sizes, and meal timing. It also allows for better management of other dietary factors such as fiber, protein, and fat intake.

By proactively planning meals, individuals with diabetes can:

1. Regulate Blood Sugar Levels: Consistent carbohydrate intake and meal timing help stabilize blood sugar levels throughout the day, preventing spikes and crashes that can occur with irregular eating patterns.

2. Manage Weight: Meal planning facilitates portion control and calorie management, making it easier to achieve and maintain a healthy weight, which is essential for diabetes management.

3. Promote Healthy Eating Habits: Planning meals in advance encourages the consumption of nutrient-dense foods such as fruits, vegetables, whole grains, lean proteins, and healthy fats, which are essential for overall health and well-being.

4. Reduce the Risk of Complications: A well-balanced diet can help reduce the risk of diabetes-related complications such as heart disease, stroke, kidney disease, and nerve damage.

Setting Goals for Meal Planning:

Before embarking on a meal planning journey, it's essential to establish clear goals that align with your individual needs, preferences, and lifestyle.

Consider the following factors when setting meal planning goals:

1. Blood Sugar Targets: Work with your healthcare provider to establish target blood sugar ranges for fasting, pre-meal, and post-meal readings. Your meal plan should aim to keep your blood sugar levels within these target ranges.

2. Weight Management Goals: Determine whether your primary goal is to lose weight, maintain your current weight, or gain weight. Adjust your meal plan accordingly to support your weight management goals.

3. Nutritional Requirements: Consider any specific dietary requirements or restrictions you may have, such as food allergies, intolerances, or cultural preferences. Ensure that your meal plan meets your nutritional needs while accommodating these factors.

4. Lifestyle Considerations: Take into account your daily schedule, work routine, social activities, and exercise regimen when planning meals. Opt for convenient and practical meal options that fit seamlessly into your lifestyle.

Understanding Portion Sizes and Carbohydrate Counting:

Portion control is a critical aspect of meal planning for individuals with diabetes. Proper portion sizes help manage calorie intake, regulate blood sugar levels, and prevent overeating. Additionally, understanding the carbohydrate content of foods is essential for individuals who need to monitor their carbohydrate intake to manage blood sugar levels effectively.

Some practical tips for portion control and carbohydrate counting:

1. Use Measuring Tools: Invest in measuring cups, spoons, and a kitchen scale to accurately measure portion sizes of foods and ingredients.

2. Learn Portion Sizes: Familiarize yourself with standard portion sizes for different food groups, such as grains, proteins, fruits, vegetables, and fats. Use visual cues or reference guides to estimate portion sizes when dining out or away from home.

3. Practice Carbohydrate Counting: Carbohydrate counting involves tracking the grams of carbohydrates consumed in each meal and snack to help manage blood sugar levels. Learn how to read food labels and identify the carbohydrate

content of various foods, including grains, fruits, starchy vegetables, dairy products, and sweets.

4. Distribute Carbohydrates Throughout the Day: Aim to distribute your carbohydrate intake evenly across meals and snacks to maintain consistent blood sugar levels throughout the day. Avoid consuming large amounts of carbohydrates in a single sitting, as this can lead to blood sugar spikes.

5. Consider the Glycemic Index: The glycemic index (GI) ranks carbohydrates based on their effect on blood sugar levels. Foods with a lower GI are digested and absorbed more slowly, resulting in gradual increases in blood sugar levels. Incorporate more low-GI foods such as whole grains, legumes, non-starchy vegetables, and fruits into your meal plan to help control blood sugar levels.

Tips for Grocery Shopping and Meal Prep:

Effective meal planning starts with a well-organized trip to the grocery store and efficient meal preparation at home. Follow these tips to streamline your grocery shopping and meal prep process:

1. Make a Shopping List: Before heading to the grocery store, create a detailed shopping list based on your planned meals and recipes. Organize your

list by food categories to ensure you don't forget any essential items.

2. Shop the Perimeter: Stick to the perimeter of the grocery store, where fresh produce, lean proteins, dairy products, and whole grains are typically located. Minimize your exposure to processed and packaged foods in the inner aisles, which tend to be higher in refined carbohydrates, sugars, and unhealthy fats.

3. Choose Fresh, Whole Foods: Prioritize fresh, whole foods such as fruits, vegetables, lean meats, poultry, fish, eggs, legumes, nuts, seeds, and whole grains. These nutrient-dense foods provide essential vitamins, minerals, fiber, and antioxidants without added sugars, sodium, or preservatives.

4. Read Food Labels: Take the time to read food labels carefully to assess the nutritional content, ingredient list, serving size, and carbohydrate content of packaged foods. Look for products with minimal added sugars, trans fats, and artificial ingredients.

5. Stock Up on Staples: Keep your pantry, refrigerator, and freezer stocked with staple ingredients such as whole grains, canned beans, frozen vegetables, herbs, spices, olive oil, vinegar, and low-sodium broth. These versatile ingredients can be used to create a variety of nutritious meals and snacks.

6. Prep Ingredients in Advance: Set aside time each week to prep and portion ingredients for meals and snacks. Wash, chop, and store fruits and vegetables for easy grab-and-go options. Cook grains, proteins, and legumes in bulk to have ready-made components for assembling meals throughout the week.

7. Utilize Meal Prep Containers: Invest in a set of meal prep containers in various sizes to portion out meals and snacks in advance. Use clear containers to easily visualize the contents and stackable containers to save space in the refrigerator or freezer.

8. Label and Date Containers: Label meal prep containers with the contents and date of preparation to keep track of freshness and avoid food waste. Use removable labels or masking tape to make it easy to update information as needed.

Getting started with meal planning for individuals newly diagnosed with diabetes requires a combination of knowledge, skills, and practical strategies. By understanding the importance of meal planning, setting clear goals, mastering portion control and carbohydrate counting, and adopting efficient grocery shopping and meal prep practices, individuals with diabetes can develop a personalized meal plan that supports their health and well-being. With dedication, consistency, and support from healthcare professionals and loved ones, meal planning can become a valuable tool for managing diabetes and improving overall quality of life.

Chapter Two

Building a Balanced Plate for Diabetes Meal Plan for Newly Diagnosed

One of the cornerstones of managing diabetes effectively is maintaining a balanced diet. For individuals who have been newly diagnosed with diabetes, understanding how to build a balanced plate is essential for controlling blood sugar levels, managing weight, and promoting overall health. In this comprehensive guide, we will explore the principles of building a balanced plate tailored specifically for individuals with diabetes.

The Importance of a Balanced Plate

A balanced plate provides the foundation for healthy eating habits and optimal diabetes management. By incorporating a variety of nutrient-rich foods in appropriate proportions, individuals with diabetes can:

1. Regulate Blood Sugar Levels: Balancing carbohydrates, proteins, and fats helps prevent blood sugar spikes and crashes, promoting stable blood sugar levels throughout the day.

2. Manage Weight: Portion control and calorie management are crucial for achieving and maintaining a healthy weight, which is essential for diabetes management and overall well-being.

3. Promote Heart Health: A balanced plate emphasizes heart-healthy foods such as fruits, vegetables, whole grains, and lean proteins, which can help reduce the risk of cardiovascular complications associated with diabetes.

4. Support Overall Health: Consuming a balanced diet provides essential nutrients, vitamins, minerals, and antioxidants that support immune function, energy production, and tissue repair, promoting overall health and vitality.

Components of a Balanced Plate

A balanced plate for individuals with diabetes should include a combination of the following components in appropriate proportions:

1. Non-Starchy Vegetables:
   - Non-starchy vegetables are low in carbohydrates and calories but rich in fiber, vitamins, and minerals.
   - Examples include leafy greens, broccoli, cauliflower, bell peppers, cucumbers, carrots, tomatoes, zucchini, and mushrooms.

- Aim to fill half of your plate with non-starchy vegetables to boost fiber intake, promote satiety, and support blood sugar control.

2. Lean Proteins:
   - Lean proteins provide essential amino acids for muscle repair and growth without excessive saturated fat and calories.
   - Examples include skinless poultry, fish, seafood, lean cuts of beef or pork, tofu, tempeh, legumes, eggs, and low-fat dairy products.
   - Include a palm-sized portion of lean protein on your plate to promote satiety, stabilize blood sugar levels, and support muscle health.

3. Whole Grains:
   - Whole grains are rich in fiber, vitamins, minerals, and complex carbohydrates that provide sustained energy and promote digestive health.
   - Examples include brown rice, quinoa, barley, oats, whole wheat bread, whole grain pasta, bulgur, and farro.
   - Limit portion sizes of whole grains to about a quarter of your plate to moderate carbohydrate intake and prevent blood sugar spikes.

4. Healthy Fats:
   - Healthy fats are essential for brain function, hormone production, and nutrient absorption, but they should be consumed in moderation.

- Examples include avocados, nuts, seeds, olive oil, canola oil, flaxseed oil, and fatty fish such as salmon, mackerel, and sardines.
- Incorporate small amounts of healthy fats into your meals to add flavor, promote satiety, and support heart health.

5. Fruits:
- Fruits are nutritious sources of vitamins, minerals, antioxidants, and natural sugars that provide energy and satisfy sweet cravings.
- Examples include berries, apples, oranges, bananas, grapes, pineapple, mango, and kiwi.
- Limit portion sizes of fruit to about a quarter of your plate and prioritize whole fruits over fruit juices or sweetened snacks to control carbohydrate intake and promote fullness.

Strategies for Building a Balanced Plate:

Building a balanced plate for diabetes meal planning involves a combination of mindful eating, portion control, and smart food choices. Here are some strategies to help you create a balanced plate:

1. Use the Plate Method: Visualize your plate as a canvas and divide it into sections to represent different food groups. Place non-starchy veggies on half of your plate, lean protein on one quarter, and whole grains or starchy vegetables on the other quarter.

2. Focus on Quality: Choose nutrient-dense foods that provide essential nutrients and support overall health. Opt for whole, minimally processed foods over refined or highly processed options whenever possible.

3. Mind Your Portions: Be mindful of portion sizes to avoid overeating and maintain calorie control. Use measuring cups, spoons, or visual cues to portion out foods according to your meal plan and nutritional goals.

4. Prioritize Fiber: Incorporate fiber-rich foods such as vegetables, fruits, whole grains, legumes, and nuts into your meals to promote satiety, regulate blood sugar levels, and support digestive health.

5. Balance Carbohydrates: Pay attention to the carbohydrate content of foods and distribute them evenly throughout the day to prevent blood sugar spikes. Choose complex carbohydrates with a low glycemic index to promote steady energy levels and minimize fluctuations in blood sugar.

6. Include Protein at Every Meal: Protein helps stabilize blood sugar levels, promote satiety, and support muscle health. Include a source of lean protein such as poultry, fish, tofu, or legumes in every meal to balance your plate and satisfy hunger.

7. Incorporate Healthy Fats: Add small amounts of healthy fats such as avocado, nuts, seeds, or olive oil to your meals to enhance flavor, promote fullness, and support nutrient absorption. Watch your portion proportions to prevent consuming too many calories.

8. Hydrate Wisely: Stay hydrated by drinking plenty of water throughout the day. Limit sugary beverages, sodas, and fruit juices, which can contribute to blood sugar spikes and unnecessary calories.

Sample Balanced Plate Meals for Diabetes:

Some examples of balanced plate meals suitable for individuals with diabetes:

1. Grilled Chicken Salad:
    - Half plate: Mixed greens, cherry tomatoes, cucumber slices, bell pepper strips
    - Quarter plate: Grilled chicken breast
    - Quarter plate: Quinoa or brown rice
    - Additional toppings: Avocado slices, almonds, vinaigrette dressing

2. Salmon with Roasted Vegetables:
    - Half plate: Roasted broccoli, cauliflower, and carrots
    - Quarter plate: Baked salmon fillet
    - Quarter plate: Quinoa or whole grain couscous

- Additional toppings: Lemon wedges, fresh herbs, olive oil drizzle

3. Vegetable Stir-Fry with Tofu:
   - Half plate: Stir-fried broccoli, bell peppers, snap peas, and mushrooms
   - Quarter plate: Stir-fried tofu or tempeh
   - Quarter plate: Brown rice or cauliflower rice
   - Additional toppings: Soy sauce, ginger, garlic, sesame oil

4. Turkey and Vegetable Skewers:
   - Half plate: Grilled zucchini, cherry tomatoes, and bell pepper skewers
   - Quarter plate: Turkey or chicken breast skewers
   - Quarter plate: Quinoa or whole wheat pita bread
   - Additional toppings: Greek yogurt tzatziki sauce, lemon wedges

5. Egg and Vegetable Omelet:
   - Half plate: Spinach, mushroom, and tomato omelet
   - Quarter plate: Whole grain toast or sweet potato hash
   - Quarter plate: Fresh mixed berries or a small fruit salad.

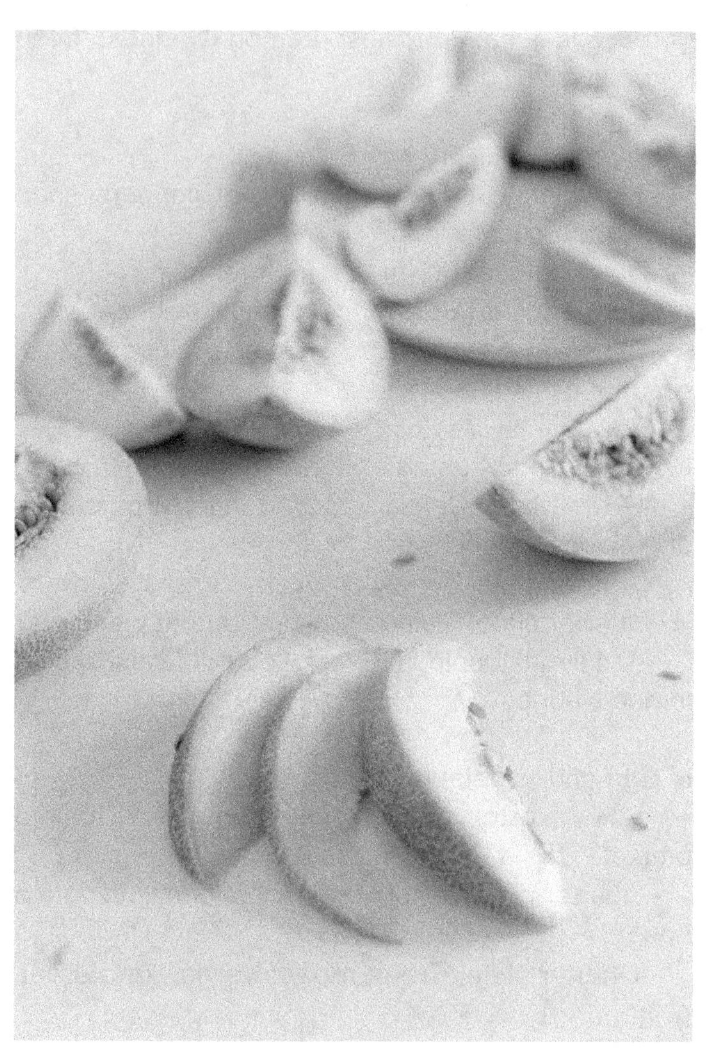

Chapter Three

Choosing The Right Foods for Diabetes Meal Plan for Newly Diagnosed

When it comes to managing diabetes, making the right food choices is essential for controlling blood sugar levels, managing weight, and preventing complications. For individuals who have been newly diagnosed with diabetes, understanding which foods to include and which to limit or avoid is crucial for successful diabetes management. In this comprehensive guide, we will explore the principles of choosing the right foods for a diabetes meal plan tailored specifically for those who are newly diagnosed.

The Importance of Choosing the Right Foods:

Choosing the right foods is the cornerstone of diabetes management. By selecting nutrient-dense, whole foods and minimizing the intake of refined carbohydrates, added sugars, unhealthy fats, and sodium, individuals with diabetes can:

1. **Regulate Blood Sugar Levels:** Certain foods have a greater impact on blood sugar levels than others. Choosing foods that are low in carbohydrates, high in fiber, and have a low glycemic index can help prevent blood sugar spikes and promote stable blood sugar levels throughout the day.

2. Manage Weight: Controlling portion sizes and selecting foods that are low in calories but high in nutrients can help individuals with diabetes achieve and maintain a healthy weight. Maintaining a healthy weight is essential for managing insulin sensitivity, blood pressure, and cholesterol levels.

3. Promote Heart Health: Diabetes is a risk factor for heart disease, so it's crucial to choose heart-healthy foods that support cardiovascular health. Opting for foods rich in omega-3 fatty acids, soluble fiber, antioxidants, and plant-based compounds can help reduce the risk of heart disease and other complications associated with diabetes.

4. Support Overall Health: A well-balanced diet that includes a variety of nutrient-rich foods provides essential vitamins, minerals, antioxidants, and phytochemicals that support immune function, energy production, tissue repair, and overall well-being. Choosing the right foods can help individuals with diabetes feel their best and live a healthy, active lifestyle.

Principles of Choosing the Right Foods:

When planning meals and snacks for diabetes management, consider the following principles to help guide your food choices:

1. Focus on Whole, Minimally Processed Foods:
   - Choose whole, minimally processed foods that are as close to their natural state as possible. These foods are typically rich in nutrients, fiber, and antioxidants and contain fewer added sugars, unhealthy fats, and sodium.
   - Examples include fruits, vegetables, whole grains, lean proteins, nuts, seeds, legumes, and dairy products with no added sugars or artificial ingredients.

2. Prioritize Non-Starchy Vegetables:

   - Non-starchy vegetables are low in carbohydrates and calories but high in fiber, vitamins, minerals, and antioxidants. They can be enjoyed in unlimited quantities and should make up a significant portion of your plate.

   - Examples include leafy greens, broccoli, cauliflower, bell peppers, cucumbers, carrots, tomatoes, zucchini, mushrooms, and asparagus.

3. Limit Refined Carbohydrates and Added Sugars:

   - Refined carbohydrates such as white bread, white rice, sugary cereals, pastries, and sugary beverages can cause rapid spikes in blood sugar levels. Limiting these foods can help stabilize blood sugar levels and reduce the risk of complications.

   - Choose whole grains such as brown rice, quinoa, oats, barley, and whole wheat bread, pasta, and crackers, which are higher in fiber and have a lower glycemic index.

4. Choose Lean Proteins:

   - Lean proteins provide essential amino acids for muscle repair and growth without excessive saturated fat and calories. Incorporate lean protein sources such as skinless poultry, fish, seafood, tofu, tempeh, legumes, eggs, and low-fat dairy products into your meals and snacks.

- Opt for grilled, baked, broiled, steamed, or roasted preparations rather than fried or breaded options to minimize added fats and calories.

5. Include Healthy Fats:

- Healthy fats are an essential part of a balanced diet and can help promote satiety, support nutrient absorption, and regulate blood sugar levels. Choose sources of healthy fats such as avocados, nuts, seeds, olive oil, fatty fish, and nut butters.

- Use moderation when adding fats to your meals and snacks, as they are calorie-dense. Aim for small portions and opt for unsaturated fats over saturated and trans fats.

6. Be Mindful of Portion Sizes:

- Portion control is key to managing calorie intake and controlling blood sugar levels. Pay attention to serving sizes and use measuring cups, spoons, or visual cues to portion out foods appropriately.

- Try to have non-starchy veggies on half of your plate, lean protein on one quarter, and whole grains or starchy vegetables on the other quarter. Add a modest amount of fruit or dairy, as well as a serving of healthy fats.

7. Read Food Labels:

- Reading food labels can help you make informed decisions about the foods you eat and identify hidden sugars, unhealthy fats, and artificial ingredients. Pay attention to serving sizes, total carbohydrate content, fiber content, and ingredient lists when choosing packaged foods.

- Look for products with minimal added sugars, trans fats, and sodium, and choose options with higher fiber content and lower glycemic index values when possible.

Examples of Right Foods for Diabetes Meal Plan:

Some examples of right foods that can be included in a diabetes meal plan for individuals who are newly diagnosed:

1. Breakfast:

- Eggs scrambled with mushrooms, tomatoes, and spinach.

- Whole grain toast or English muffin with avocado spread

- On the side, some sliced melon or fresh berries.

- Unsweetened almond milk or Greek yogurt with nuts and seeds

2. Lunch:
   - Grilled chicken or tofu salad with mixed greens, cucumber, bell peppers, and chickpeas
   - Quinoa or brown rice pilaf with roasted vegetables
   - Olive oil and vinegar dressing or hummus as a topping
   - Apple slices or carrot sticks for crunch

3. Dinner:
   - Baked salmon or tofu with asparagus, broccoli, and cauliflower
   - Quinoa or whole grain pasta with marinara sauce and sautéed spinach
   - Mixed green salad with cherry tomatoes, avocado, and balsamic vinaigrette
   - Fresh fruit salad or Greek yogurt for dessert

4. Snacks:
   - Greek yogurt paired with almonds and berries
- Apple slices with almond or peanut butter; - Hummus with carrot sticks or cucumber slices.
   - Air-popped popcorn seasoned with herbs and spices

- Cottage cheese with pineapple or peach slices

Choosing the right foods is essential for individuals who have been newly diagnosed with diabetes. By focusing on whole, minimally processed foods; prioritizing non-starchy vegetables; limiting refined carbohydrates and added sugars; choosing lean proteins and healthy fats; being mindful of portion sizes; and reading food labels, individuals with diabetes can create a balanced meal plan that supports blood sugar control, weight management, and overall health. With dedication, consistency, and support from healthcare professionals and loved ones, making the right food choices can become second nature and contribute to a healthier, happier life with diabetes.

Chapter Four

Meal Planning for Different Lifestyles

Meal planning is not a one-size-fits-all approach, especially when it comes to managing diabetes. Different lifestyles require unique strategies for meal planning to accommodate individual preferences, cultural backgrounds, dietary restrictions, and health goals. For individuals who have been newly diagnosed with diabetes, understanding how to adapt their meal plan to fit their lifestyle is essential for successful diabetes management. In this comprehensive guide, we will explore various lifestyles and provide practical tips for meal planning tailored to each lifestyle for newly diagnosed individuals with diabetes.

1. **Busy Lifestyles:**

For individuals with busy lifestyles, meal planning is crucial for maintaining healthy eating habits amidst hectic schedules. Here are some strategies for meal planning for busy individuals with diabetes:

- Batch Cooking: Dedicate one day a week to prepare large batches of meals and portion them into individual servings for quick and easy meals throughout the week.
- Pre-cut and Pre-packaged Foods: Purchase pre-cut fruits and vegetables, pre-cooked grains, and pre-packaged lean proteins to streamline meal preparation and save time.
- One-Pot Meals: Prepare simple and nutritious one-pot meals such as soups, stews, stir-fries, and casseroles that can be made in large batches and reheated as needed.
- Grab-and-Go Options: Stock up on healthy grab-and-go options such as fresh fruit, Greek yogurt, nuts, seeds, whole grain crackers, and pre-made salads for convenient snacks and meals on the run.

2. **Vegetarian and Vegan Lifestyles**:

Vegetarian and vegan lifestyles can be compatible with diabetes management with proper meal planning. Here are some tips for incorporating vegetarian and vegan options into a diabetes meal plan:

- Plant-Based Proteins: Include a variety of plant-based protein sources such as tofu, tempeh, edamame, lentils, beans, chickpeas, quinoa, nuts, and seeds to meet protein needs and promote satiety.

- Colorful Vegetables: Fill your plate with a colorful array of non-starchy vegetables such as leafy greens, bell peppers, broccoli, cauliflower, carrots, tomatoes, and zucchini to boost fiber intake and control blood sugar levels.

- Whole Grains: Choose whole grains such as brown rice, quinoa, barley, oats, bulgur, and whole wheat pasta to provide sustained energy and promote digestive health.

- Healthy Fats: Incorporate sources of healthy fats such as avocados, nuts, seeds, olive oil, and coconut oil into your meals to add flavor, texture, and satiety.

3. **Cultural Preferences**:

For individuals with specific cultural preferences or dietary traditions, adapting a diabetes meal plan may require creativity and flexibility. Here are some tips for incorporating cultural preferences into a diabetes meal plan:

- Traditional Recipes: Modify traditional recipes to make them diabetes-friendly by using healthier cooking methods, reducing added sugars and unhealthy fats, and incorporating more vegetables and whole grains.

- Cultural Staples: Identify cultural staples that align with diabetes management goals, such as beans, lentils, whole grains, vegetables, lean proteins, and herbs and spices, and incorporate them into your meals regularly.

- Family Favorites: Involve family members in meal planning and preparation to ensure that diabetes-friendly meals are enjoyed by everyone. Experiment with new recipes and flavors to find healthy alternatives to family favorites.

- Cultural Celebrations: Plan ahead for cultural celebrations and holidays by modifying traditional dishes to make them diabetes-friendly or offering healthier alternatives. Focus on portion control and balance to enjoy traditional foods in moderation.

4. **Low-Income Lifestyles:**

Managing diabetes on a limited budget can be challenging, but with careful planning and resourcefulness, it is possible to eat healthily without breaking the bank. Some tips for meal planning on a budget:

- Shop Smart: Look for sales, discounts, and coupons to save money on groceries. Compare prices and buy in bulk when possible to get the most value for your money.
- Plan Meals in Advance: Plan your meals for the week based on what's on sale and what you already have on hand. Creatively use leftovers to minimize food waste and stretch your food budget.
- Buy Affordable Staples: Focus on affordable staples such as beans, lentils, rice, pasta, potatoes, eggs, canned vegetables, frozen fruits and vegetables, and generic brands to save money without sacrificing nutrition.
- Cook at Home: Prepare meals at home rather than eating out or buying pre-packaged convenience foods, which are often more expensive and less nutritious. Cooking from scratch allows you to control the ingredients and portion sizes.

5. **Gluten-Free Lifestyles:**

For individuals with celiac disease or gluten intolerance, following a gluten-free diet is essential for managing symptoms and preventing complications. Here are some tips for meal planning for a gluten-free lifestyle:

- Focus on Naturally Gluten-Free Foods: Emphasize naturally gluten-free foods such as fruits, vegetables, lean proteins, dairy products, nuts, seeds, legumes, and gluten-free whole grains like quinoa, rice, millet, and buckwheat.

- Read Labels Carefully: When shopping for packaged or processed foods, always read labels carefully to identify gluten-containing ingredients such as wheat, barley, rye, and their derivatives. Seek out labels that are certified gluten-free to make sure the food is safe to eat.

- Explore Gluten-Free Alternatives: Experiment with gluten-free alternatives for your favorite dishes, such as using gluten-free flour blends for baking, corn or rice-based pasta, and gluten-free bread or wraps made from alternative grains like sorghum or almond flour.

- Be Mindful of Cross-Contamination: Avoid cross-contamination by using separate utensils, cutting boards, and kitchen appliances for gluten-free cooking. Clean surfaces thoroughly and be cautious when dining out to prevent accidental exposure to gluten.

- Plan Ahead for Meals and Snacks: Take time to plan meals and snacks in advance to ensure you have gluten-free options readily available. Pack gluten-free snacks for on-the-go convenience and prepare meals using fresh, whole ingredients whenever possible.

- Seek Gluten-Free Resources and Support: Connect with support groups, online forums, and healthcare professionals specializing in gluten-free nutrition to gather information, share experiences, and access valuable resources for maintaining a gluten-free lifestyle.

- Communicate Dietary Needs: When dining out or attending social gatherings, communicate your dietary needs to restaurant staff or hosts in advance to ensure gluten-free options are available. Never be afraid to inquire about menu items and food preparation techniques.

- Monitor Symptoms and Adjust Accordingly: Keep track of any symptoms or reactions to food and make adjustments to your diet as needed. Work closely with healthcare providers to manage symptoms and optimize your gluten-free lifestyle.

Transitioning to a gluten-free lifestyle requires diligence, patience, and creativity, but with the right knowledge and support, it can become a rewarding and empowering journey towards improved health and well-being. Embrace the diversity of gluten-free foods and discover delicious ways to enjoy a fulfilling and satisfying diet without gluten-containing ingredients.

Chapter Five

Managing Special Occasions and Dining Out

Special occasions and dining out can present unique challenges for individuals who have been newly diagnosed with diabetes. From navigating unfamiliar menus to resisting tempting treats, managing blood sugar levels while enjoying social gatherings can be a balancing act. However, with careful planning, mindfulness, and a few smart strategies, individuals with diabetes can successfully navigate special occasions and dining out while adhering to their meal plan. In this comprehensive guide, we will explore practical tips and strategies for managing special occasions and dining out for newly diagnosed individuals with diabetes.

1. **Planning Ahead**:

The key to successfully managing special occasions and dining out with diabetes is planning ahead. By taking proactive steps to prepare for these situations, individuals can minimize stress and ensure they stay on track with their diabetes management goals. Some tips for planning ahead:

-Check the Menu in Advance: If possible, review the menu of the restaurant or event venue ahead of time to identify diabetes-friendly options and plan your meal accordingly. Look for grilled or baked protein options, salads with lean protein, and vegetable-based dishes.
-Communicate with Hosts or Restaurants: If attending a special event or dining out at a restaurant, don't hesitate to communicate your dietary needs and preferences to the hosts or restaurant staff. They may be able to accommodate special requests or provide information about ingredient substitutions.
-Bring a Diabetes-Friendly Dish: Offer to bring a diabetes-friendly dish to share at social gatherings to ensure there are nutritious options available. Choose dishes that are low in carbohydrates, sugar-free, and high in fiber and protein.
-Pack Snacks: Carry diabetes-friendly snacks with you when attending special occasions or dining out to prevent blood sugar fluctuations and avoid overindulging in unhealthy options. Portable options such as nuts, seeds, fruit,

cheese, and whole grain crackers are convenient choices.

-Stay Hydrated: Throughout the day, sip on lots of water to stay hydrated and manage cravings and hunger. Opt for water, unsweetened tea, or sparkling water with lemon or lime instead of sugary beverages or alcoholic drinks.

2. **Making Smart Choices**:

When faced with a variety of tempting food options at special occasions or restaurants, making smart choices is essential for managing blood sugar levels and staying on track with your diabetes meal plan.
Here are some strategies for making smart choices:

-Focus on Portions: Practice portion control by sticking to appropriate serving sizes and avoiding oversized portions. Use visual cues or portion control tools to help estimate serving sizes if necessary.
-Eat A Lot of veggies: Make sure that non-starchy veggies like leafy greens, broccoli, cauliflower, peppers, and cucumbers make up half of your meal. Vegetables are low in calories and carbohydrates but high in fiber, vitamins, and minerals, making them an

excellent choice for managing blood sugar levels.

-Choose Lean Proteins: Opt for lean protein options such as grilled chicken, fish, tofu, or legumes to help stabilize blood sugar levels and promote satiety. Limit intake of processed meats, fried foods, and fatty cuts of meat, which can be high in saturated fat and sodium.

-Select Whole Grains: Choose whole grain options such as brown rice, quinoa, barley, or whole wheat bread instead of refined grains like white rice or white bread. Whole grains are higher in fiber and nutrients and have a lower glycemic index, which can help prevent blood sugar spikes.

-Limit Added Sugars: Be mindful of hidden sources of added sugars in sauces, dressings, marinades, and condiments. Choose options with little or no added sugars and use sparingly to avoid unnecessary spikes in blood sugar levels.

-Be Mindful of Alcohol Intake: If choosing to consume alcoholic beverages, do so in moderation and be mindful of their impact on blood sugar levels. Opt for light beer, dry wines, or spirits mixed with calorie-free mixers instead of sugary cocktails or sweetened drinks.

3. **Managing Desserts and Treats**:

Special occasions often involve indulging in desserts and treats, which can pose challenges for individuals with diabetes. However, with moderation and careful planning, it is possible to enjoy sweet treats while managing blood sugar levels effectively. Here are some tips for managing desserts and treats:

- Choose Wisely: Be selective about which desserts and treats you indulge in and opt for smaller portions of your favorites. Choose desserts that are lower in sugar and higher in fiber, such as fruit-based desserts or desserts made with whole grains.
-Practice Portion Control: Enjoying a small serving of dessert can satisfy cravings without causing significant blood sugar spikes. Use portion control techniques such as sharing desserts with others, splitting desserts in half, or using smaller plates or bowls.
-Make Substitutions: Look for healthier alternatives or make ingredient substitutions to reduce the sugar and carbohydrate content of desserts. For example, use sugar substitutes, whole grain flours, and unsweetened

applesauce instead of sugar, refined flour, and butter in recipes.

-Savor Mindfully: Take the time to savor and enjoy each bite of dessert mindfully, paying attention to taste, texture, and aroma. Eating slowly can help you appreciate the flavors and feel satisfied with smaller portions.

-Balance with Protein and Fiber: Pairing desserts with protein and fiber-rich foods can help slow down the absorption of sugar into the bloodstream and prevent blood sugar spikes. Enjoy dessert with a serving of Greek yogurt, cottage cheese, or nuts for added protein and fiber.

4. **Staying Active**:

Regular physical activity is an essential component of diabetes management and can help offset the effects of indulging in special occasion foods or dining out. Incorporating physical activity into your routine can help lower blood sugar levels, improve insulin sensitivity, and promote overall health and well-being.

Here are some tips for staying active:

-Plan Ahead: Schedule physical activity before or after special occasions or dining out to help offset the effects of indulging in high-calorie or high-carbohydrate foods. On most days of the week, try to get in at least 30 minutes of moderate-intensity aerobic exercise, including brisk walking, cycling, or swimming.

-Be Flexible: If you're unable to stick to your regular exercise routine due to special events or dining out, be flexible and find alternative ways to stay active. Incorporate short bursts of physical activity throughout the day, such as taking the stairs, walking during breaks, or doing quick home workouts.

-Stay Active Together: Invite friends or family members to join you in physical activities such as walking, hiking, dancing, or playing sports. Exercising with others can provide motivation, accountability, and social support, making it more enjoyable and sustainable.

-Focus on Enjoyment: Choose physical activities that you enjoy and look forward to doing. Whether it's dancing to your favorite music, practicing yoga, or playing a sport, finding activities that bring you joy can make exercise feel less like a chore and more like a fun part of your daily routine.

5. **Managing Stress:**

Special occasions and dining out can sometimes be stressful, especially for individuals with diabetes who are trying to manage their blood sugar levels effectively. Managing stress is essential for maintaining overall health and well-being and can help prevent emotional eating and blood sugar fluctuations.
Here are some tips for managing stress:

-Practice Relaxation Techniques: Incorporate relaxation techniques such as deep breathing, meditation, yoga, or progressive muscle relaxation into your daily routine to help reduce stress levels and promote a sense of calmness.
-Stay Active: Engage in regular physical activity to release endorphins and combat stress. Choose activities you enjoy, such as walking, swimming, dancing, or cycling, and make time for exercise as part of your self-care routine.
-Prioritize Sleep: Aim for adequate and restful sleep each night to support overall well-being and resilience to stress. Create a relaxing bedtime routine, minimize screen time before

bed, and ensure your sleep environment is comfortable and conducive to rest.

-Set Realistic Expectations: Manage expectations for special occasions and dining out by setting realistic goals and priorities. Focus on enjoying the experience rather than striving for perfection in blood sugar management.

-Plan Ahead: Prepare for special occasions or dining out by checking menus in advance, communicating dietary needs to hosts or restaurant staff, and bringing diabetes-friendly snacks if needed. Planning ahead can reduce anxiety and help you make informed choices.

-Seek Support: Reach out to friends, family members, or a healthcare professional for emotional support and guidance. Speaking with someone about your worries and emotions helps reduce tension and give you perspective.

-Practice Mindful Eating: Be present and mindful during meals, savoring each bite and paying attention to hunger and fullness cues. When eating, stay away from stressful conversations or screens.

-Use Positive Coping Strategies: Develop positive coping strategies such as journaling, engaging in hobbies, listening to music, or spending time in nature to manage stress and boost mood.

-Learn to Say No: Set boundaries and prioritize self-care by learning to say no to commitments or activities that contribute to stress or overwhelm.

- Stay Flexible: Embrace flexibility and adaptability in managing diabetes during special occasions. If unexpected challenges arise, focus on problem-solving and making adjustments rather than dwelling on setbacks.

By implementing these stress management techniques, individuals with diabetes can navigate special occasions and dining out with greater ease and enjoyment while maintaining optimal blood sugar levels and overall well-being. Remember, managing stress is a valuable skill that supports healthy lifestyle choices and empowers individuals to thrive despite the challenges of diabetes management.

Chapter Six

Snacking Smart

Snacking plays a significant role in managing blood sugar levels, hunger, and energy levels throughout the day, especially for individuals who have been newly diagnosed with diabetes. However, snacking can also present challenges, as it's essential to choose snacks that are balanced, nutritious, and compatible with diabetes management goals. In this comprehensive guide, we will explore the principles of snacking smart for individuals who are newly diagnosed with diabetes, providing practical tips, delicious snack ideas, and strategies for incorporating healthy snacks into a diabetes meal plan.

The Role of Snacking in Diabetes Management:

Snacking can serve several purposes for individuals with diabetes, including:

1. Blood Sugar Control: Smart snacking can help prevent blood sugar fluctuations between

meals by providing a steady source of carbohydrates, protein, and healthy fats.

2. Hunger Management: Well-planned snacks can help curb hunger and prevent overeating at mealtime, promoting portion control and weight management.

3. Energy Boost: Healthy snacks can provide a quick energy boost and combat fatigue, helping individuals stay alert and focused throughout the day.

4. Nutrient Intake: Snacks can be an opportunity to incorporate additional nutrients, vitamins, and minerals into the diet, supporting overall health and well-being.

Principles of Snacking Smart with Diabetes:

When snacking with diabetes, it's essential to follow these principles to make healthy choices and support blood sugar control:

1. Choose Nutrient-Dense Foods: Opt for snacks that are rich in nutrients, such as vitamins, minerals, fiber, and antioxidants. Focus on whole, minimally processed foods that provide sustained energy and promote satiety.

2. Balance Carbohydrates with Protein and Healthy Fats: Aim to include a combination of carbohydrates, protein, and healthy fats in each snack to help stabilize blood sugar levels and promote fullness. This combination can help slow down the absorption of sugar into the bloodstream and prevent blood sugar spikes.

3. Control Portion Sizes: Be mindful of portion sizes when snacking to avoid overeating and consuming excess calories. Use measuring cups, spoons, or visual cues to portion out snacks appropriately according to your meal plan and nutritional goals.

4. Be Mindful of Timing: Space out snacks evenly throughout the day to prevent prolonged periods of hunger and maintain steady blood sugar levels. Aim to snack every 3-4 hours between meals to keep energy levels stable and prevent overeating at mealtime.

5. Stay Hydrated: Drink plenty of water throughout the day, especially when snacking, to stay hydrated and help control hunger and cravings. Choose water, herbal tea, or sparkling water with lemon or lime over sugary beverages or fruit juices.

Smart Snack Ideas for Diabetes

Here are some delicious and nutritious snack ideas for individuals who are newly diagnosed with diabetes:

1. **Greek Yogurt Parfait**:
     - Simple Greek yogurt adorned with a sprinkling of nuts or seeds, a drizzle of honey, or a pinch of cinnamon, and fresh berries.
   - Greek yogurt provides protein and calcium, while berries add fiber and antioxidants for blood sugar control.

2. **Vegetable Sticks with Hummus**:
   - Sliced cucumber, carrot sticks, bell pepper strips, and cherry tomatoes served with a side of hummus for dipping.
   - Hummus is a good source of plant-based protein and healthy fats, while vegetables provide fiber and essential nutrients.

3. **Apple Slices with Peanut Butter**:
     - Apple slices paired with natural peanut butter or almond butter for a satisfying sweet and savory snack.
   - Apples are rich in fiber, while nut butter provides protein and healthy fats to keep you feeling full and satisfied.

4. **Hard-Boiled Eggs with Whole Grain Crackers:**

- Hard-boiled eggs served with whole grain crackers or rice cakes for a portable and protein-rich snack.

- Eggs are a complete source of protein, while whole grain crackers provide complex carbohydrates for sustained energy.

5. **Cottage Cheese with Pineapple**:

- Low-fat cottage cheese topped with diced pineapple or mixed fruit for a refreshing and protein-packed snack.

- Pineapple offers natural sweetness and vitamin C, while cottage cheese is rich in calcium and protein.

6. **Nut and dried fruit trail mix:**

- Homemade trail mix made with a mix of nuts (such as almonds, walnuts, and cashews) and dried fruit (such as raisins, apricots, and cranberries).

- Nuts are rich in protein and healthy fats, while dried fruit adds natural sweetness and fiber for sustained energy.

7. **Edamame with Sea Salt**:
   - Steamed edamame sprinkled with sea salt for a crunchy and satisfying snack.
   - Edamame is a good source of plant-based protein and fiber, making it an excellent option for blood sugar control.

8. **Avocado Toast with Whole Grain Bread:**
   - Whole grain toast topped with mashed avocado, cherry tomatoes, and a sprinkle of feta cheese or everything bagel seasoning.
   - Avocado provides healthy fats and fiber, while whole grain bread adds complex carbohydrates for lasting energy.

Strategies for Snacking Smart While Dining Out:

Dining out can present challenges for individuals with diabetes, but with a little planning and mindfulness, it's possible to make healthy choices while enjoying restaurant meals. Here are some strategies for snacking smart while dining out:

1. Check the Menu in Advance: Review the restaurant's menu online before dining out to identify diabetes-friendly options and plan your meal accordingly. Look for grilled or baked

protein options, salads with lean protein, and vegetable-based dishes.

2. Ask for Modifications: Don't hesitate to ask your server for modifications or substitutions to make dishes more diabetes-friendly. Request grilled or steamed vegetables instead of fried sides, dressings on the side, and whole grain or vegetable-based alternatives to refined carbohydrates.

3. Control Portion Sizes: Be mindful of portion sizes when dining out and avoid oversized portions by sharing dishes with a dining companion or asking for a to-go box to save half for later. Stick to appropriate serving sizes to prevent overeating and blood sugar spikes.

4. Be Mindful of Sauces and Condiments: Be aware of hidden sources of added sugars, unhealthy fats, and sodium in sauces, dressings, marinades, and condiments. Ask for sauces and dressings on the side and use sparingly to control calories and blood sugar levels.

5. Choose Water or Unsweetened Beverages: Opt for water, unsweetened tea, or sparkling water with lemon or lime instead of sugary

beverages or alcoholic drinks. Drinking calorie-free beverages can help control hunger and prevent unnecessary calorie consumption.

Snacking smart is an essential component of diabetes management for individuals who have been newly diagnosed with the condition. By following the principles of snacking smart, choosing balanced and nutritious snacks, and incorporating smart snacking strategies into daily life, individuals with diabetes can maintain stable blood sugar levels, manage hunger and cravings, and support overall health and well-being. With a little planning, mindfulness, and creativity, snacking can be an enjoyable and satisfying part of a diabetes meal plan, helping individuals stay on track with their diabetes management goals and live their best lives with diabetes.

Chapter Seven

Understanding Labels and Nutrition Facts

Navigating food labels and nutrition facts is essential for individuals who have been newly diagnosed with diabetes. Understanding how to interpret food labels can empower individuals to make informed and healthy choices that support blood sugar control, weight management, and overall health. In this comprehensive guide, we will explore the basics of food labels and nutrition facts, providing practical tips and insights for incorporating label reading into a diabetes meal plan.

Why Understanding Labels Matters

Reading food labels is crucial for individuals with diabetes for several reasons:

1. Portion Control: Understanding serving sizes and portion information on food labels helps individuals manage their carbohydrate intake, which directly impacts blood sugar levels.

2. Nutrient Content: Examining the nutrient content of foods helps individuals make choices that align with their dietary goals, such as limiting sugar, sodium, and unhealthy fats while prioritizing fiber, vitamins, and minerals.

3. Ingredient Awareness: Checking ingredient lists allows individuals to identify hidden sources of added sugars, unhealthy fats, and artificial additives, which can impact blood sugar levels and overall health.

4. Comparing Products: Reading labels enables individuals to compare similar products and choose the ones that best fit their nutritional needs and preferences.

Key Components of Food Labels

Understanding food labels involves knowing how to interpret different components accurately. Here are the key components typically found on food labels:

1. Serving Size: This indicates the recommended portion size of the food or beverage and the number of servings per package. All other nutrition information on the label is based on this serving size.

2. Calories: The number of calories per serving gives an indication of the energy content of the food. Managing calorie intake is essential for weight management and overall health.

3. Total Carbohydrates: This includes all carbohydrates, including sugars, fiber, and starches. For individuals with diabetes, monitoring total carbohydrates is crucial for managing blood sugar levels.

4. Dietary fiber: The body is unable to digest fiber, a form of carbohydrate. High-fiber foods can help stabilize blood sugar levels and promote digestive health.

5. Sugars: This indicates the amount of naturally occurring and added sugars in the product. It's important for individuals with diabetes to limit added sugars to prevent blood sugar spikes.

6. Protein: Protein is essential for muscle repair and growth. Including adequate protein in meals and snacks helps promote satiety and stabilize blood sugar levels.

7. Total Fat: This includes both healthy fats (unsaturated fats) and unhealthy fats (saturated and trans fats). Choosing foods low in unhealthy fats supports heart health and overall well-being.

8. Saturated Fat and Trans Fat: These types of fats can raise cholesterol levels and increase the risk of heart disease. Limiting saturated and trans fats is recommended for individuals with diabetes.

9. Sodium: This indicates the amount of salt in the product. Consuming too much sodium can lead to high blood pressure, so it's important to choose low-sodium options whenever possible.

Tips for Reading Food Labels

To make the most of food labels and nutrition facts, consider these practical tips:

1. Start with the Serving Size: Always check the serving size listed on the label and compare it to the portion you intend to consume. This helps avoid overeating and accurately assess nutrient intake.

2. Focus on Total Carbohydrates: Pay close attention to the total carbohydrates, especially sugars and fiber. Aim for foods that are higher in fiber and lower in added sugars to help control blood sugar levels.

3. Look for Whole Ingredients: Choose foods with simple and recognizable ingredients. Avoid products with long ingredient lists full of artificial additives, preservatives, and sweeteners.

4. Check the % Daily Value (%DV): The %DV indicates how much of a specific nutrient (such as fat, sodium, or fiber) one serving of the food provides based on a 2,000-calorie diet. Use %DV to assess the nutritional value of foods and make comparisons between products.

5. Be Aware of Hidden Sugars: Learn to identify hidden sources of added sugars by checking the ingredient list for terms like sucrose, high-fructose corn syrup, agave nectar, and cane sugar.

6. Compare Similar Products: When choosing between similar products, compare labels to select the one with lower amounts of sugar,

saturated fat, and sodium, and higher amounts of fiber and protein.

7. Consider Nutrient Density: Choose foods that are nutrient-dense, meaning they provide a high amount of vitamins, minerals, and other beneficial nutrients relative to their calorie content.

Interpreting Common Label Claims:

Food labels often include various claims and certifications that can influence purchasing decisions. Here's how to interpret some common label claims:

1. "Sugar-Free": This means the product contains less than 0.5 grams of sugar per serving. However, it may still contain carbohydrates from other sources.

2. "Low Sodium": This indicates that the product contains 140 milligrams or less of sodium per serving, making it suitable for individuals watching their sodium intake.

3. "Whole Grain": Look for products labeled "100% whole grain" or "100% whole wheat" to

ensure they contain whole grains rather than refined grains.

4. "Low-Fat" or "Fat-Free": These labels indicate that the product contains reduced or minimal amounts of fat. However, be mindful of added sugars and artificial ingredients used to enhance flavor.

5. "Organic": Foods labeled as organic are produced without synthetic pesticides, herbicides, or genetically modified organisms (GMOs). Organic certification ensures higher standards of environmental sustainability and animal welfare.

Understanding labels and nutrition facts is a valuable skill for individuals who have been newly diagnosed with diabetes. By learning how to interpret food labels, compare products, and make informed choices based on nutritional information, individuals can better manage their blood sugar levels, support overall health, and achieve their diabetes management goals. Incorporating label reading into a diabetes meal plan empowers individuals to take control of their dietary choices and make choices that align with their health and wellness objectives. With practice and awareness, navigating food labels becomes second nature, leading to improved dietary habits and better long-term outcomes for individuals living with diabetes.

Chapter Eight

Managing Blood Sugar Levels Through Diet

Properly managing blood sugar levels is crucial for individuals who have been newly diagnosed with diabetes. Diet plays a fundamental role in diabetes management, as certain foods can directly impact blood sugar levels. By adopting a balanced and tailored meal plan, individuals with diabetes can achieve better control over their blood sugar levels, promote overall health, and reduce the risk of complications. In this comprehensive guide, we will explore the principles of managing blood sugar levels through diet, providing practical tips, meal ideas, and strategies for incorporating healthy eating into a diabetes meal plan.

Understanding Blood Sugar Levels

Blood sugar levels, also known as blood glucose levels, refer to the amount of sugar (glucose) present in the bloodstream. Glucose is a vital source of energy for the body's cells and organs. However, individuals with diabetes have difficulty regulating blood sugar levels due to either insufficient insulin production (Type 1 diabetes) or insulin resistance (Type 2 diabetes).

Monitoring and managing blood sugar levels is essential for individuals with diabetes to prevent hyperglycemia (high blood sugar) and hypoglycemia (low blood sugar) episodes, both of which can have adverse effects on health and well-being.

Principles of Managing Blood Sugar Levels Through Diet

1. Balancing Carbohydrates: Carbohydrates have the most significant impact on blood sugar levels because they break down into glucose during digestion. However, not all carbohydrates are equal. Focus on choosing complex carbohydrates (such as whole grains, fruits, vegetables, and legumes) over simple carbohydrates (such as sugars and refined grains) to minimize blood sugar spikes.

2. Prioritizing Fiber: Fiber is a type of carbohydrate that the body cannot digest. High-fiber foods help slow down the absorption of glucose into the bloodstream, promoting more stable blood sugar levels. Incorporate

plenty of fiber-rich foods like vegetables, fruits, whole grains, nuts, and seeds into your diet.

3. Including Lean Proteins: Protein helps stabilize blood sugar levels and promote satiety. Include lean protein sources such as poultry, fish, tofu, legumes, and low-fat dairy in your meals and snacks.

4. Choosing Healthy Fats: Incorporate heart-healthy fats such as avocados, nuts, seeds, olive oil, and fatty fish (like salmon and mackerel) into your diet. Good fats lower the risk of heart disease and enhance insulin sensitivity.

5. Monitoring Portion Sizes: Controlling portion sizes is crucial for managing blood sugar levels. Avoid overeating and practice portion control by using smaller plates, measuring food portions, and being mindful of serving sizes.

6. Timing Meals and Snacks: Eat regular meals and snacks throughout the day to prevent blood sugar fluctuations. Aim for consistent carbohydrate intake spaced evenly throughout the day to maintain stable blood sugar levels.

7. Limiting Added Sugars and Processed Foods: Minimize consumption of foods and beverages high in added sugars, such as sugary drinks, desserts, candies, and sweetened snacks. Opt for whole, minimally processed foods to support blood sugar control.

Useful Advice for Controlling Blood Sugar Levels with Diet

1. Create a Balanced Plate: Use the plate method to portion out your meals: Fill half of your plate with non-starchy vegetables (like leafy greens, broccoli, and bell peppers), one-quarter with lean protein (such as chicken, fish, or tofu), and one-quarter with whole grains or starchy vegetables (like brown rice, quinoa, or sweet potatoes).

2. Choose Whole Grains: Opt for whole grains over refined grains to provide sustained energy and prevent blood sugar spikes. Examples of whole grains include oats, barley, quinoa, bulgur, and whole wheat products.

3. Incorporate Plenty of Vegetables: Vegetables are low in calories and carbohydrates but high in fiber, vitamins, and

minerals. Aim to include a variety of colorful vegetables in your meals and snacks to promote overall health and blood sugar control.

4. Snack Smart: Choose diabetes-friendly snacks that combine protein and fiber to help stabilize blood sugar levels between meals. Avoid sugary snacks and opt for options like Greek yogurt with berries, raw vegetables with hummus, or a handful of nuts.

5. Read Food Labels: Check food labels for total carbohydrate content, serving sizes, and added sugars. Pay attention to portion sizes and be mindful of hidden sources of sugar and unhealthy fats in packaged foods.

Sample Meal Plan for Managing Blood Sugar Levels

Here's a sample meal plan that demonstrates how to manage blood sugar levels through diet:

Breakfast:
- Spinach and feta omelet made with egg whites and served with whole grain toast
- Sliced tomatoes and cucumbers
- Unsweetened herbal tea or black coffee

Mid-Morning Snack:
-Nuts and seeds sprinkled over Greek yogurt

Lunch:
- Grilled chicken salad with mixed greens, cherry tomatoes, cucumbers, and avocado
- Quinoa pilaf with chickpeas
- Sparkling water with lemon or lime

Afternoon Snack:
- Carrot sticks with hummus

Dinner:
- Baked salmon with lemon and dill
- Roasted Brussels sprouts and carrots
- Brown rice pilaf
- Sparkling water or herbal tea

Evening Snack:
- Apple slices with almond butter

Strategies for Dining Out and Special Occasions

Managing blood sugar levels while dining out or attending special occasions requires planning and preparation. Here are some strategies:

1. Review Menus in Advance: Check restaurant menus online ahead of time to identify diabetes-friendly options. Look for grilled or baked protein dishes, salads, and vegetable-based sides.

2. Ask for Modifications: Don't hesitate to ask for modifications at restaurants, such as substituting vegetables for fries or requesting dressings and sauces on the side.

3. Practice Portion Control: Control portion sizes by sharing dishes, ordering appetizers as entrees, or requesting a to-go box to save leftovers.

4. Choose Smart Beverages: Opt for water, unsweetened tea, or sparkling water with lemon or lime instead of sugary beverages or alcoholic drinks.

5. Plan Ahead for Special Occasions: Bring a diabetes-friendly dish to share at gatherings, and communicate your dietary needs with hosts to ensure there are suitable options available.

Managing blood sugar levels through diet is essential for individuals who have been newly diagnosed with diabetes. By adopting a balanced and nutritious meal plan that focuses on complex carbohydrates, lean proteins, healthy fats, and plenty of vegetables, individuals with diabetes can achieve better blood sugar control, promote overall health, and reduce the risk of complications. Incorporating practical tips, meal ideas, and strategies for dining out and special occasions empowers individuals to make informed choices and take control of their diabetes management. With dedication, knowledge, and support, managing blood sugar levels through diet becomes an integral part of a healthy and fulfilling lifestyle for individuals living with diabetes.

Chapter Nine

Exercise and Meal Planning

Physical activity is a cornerstone of diabetes management, complementing meal planning to support overall health and blood sugar control. For individuals who are newly diagnosed with diabetes, understanding how exercise impacts meal planning and vice versa is crucial for achieving optimal health outcomes. In this comprehensive guide, we will explore the relationship between exercise and meal planning, providing practical insights, strategies, and meal ideas to empower individuals in their diabetes journey.

The Role of Exercise in Diabetes Management

There are many advantages to regular exercise for those with diabetes:

1. Blood Sugar Control: Physical activity helps lower blood sugar levels by increasing insulin sensitivity, allowing cells to use glucose more effectively.
2. Weight Management: Exercise promotes weight loss or maintenance, reducing insulin

resistance and improving blood sugar regulation.

3. Heart Health: Physical activity lowers the risk of heart disease, a common complication of diabetes.

4. Stress Reduction: Exercise reduces stress levels, which can affect blood sugar levels.

5. Improved Overall Well-being: Regular exercise enhances mood, boosts energy levels, and promotes better sleep quality.

Types of Exercise for Diabetes

Various types of exercise benefit individuals with diabetes:

1. Aerobic Exercise: Activities like walking, cycling, swimming, and dancing improve cardiovascular health and aid in blood sugar control.

2. Strength Training: Resistance exercises using weights or body weight increase muscle mass, improve insulin sensitivity, and enhance metabolism.

3. Flexibility and Balance Exercises: Stretching, yoga, and tai chi improve flexibility, balance, and overall mobility.

Exercise Guidelines for Diabetes:

The American Diabetes Association (ADA) recommends the following exercise guidelines for individuals with diabetes:

1. 150 Minutes per Week: Aim for at least 150 minutes of moderate-intensity aerobic exercise spread across most days of the week.
2. Resistance Training: Perform strength training exercises on two or more days per week.
3. Flexibility and Balance Exercises: Include flexibility and balance activities regularly.

How Exercise Impacts Meal Planning

Exercise influences meal planning in several ways:

1. Carbohydrate Intake: Adjust carbohydrate intake based on the duration and intensity of exercise. Increase carbohydrates before prolonged or intense workouts to provide fuel for muscles.
2. Timing of Meals: Time meals and snacks around exercise sessions to prevent blood sugar fluctuations. Before working out, eat a well-balanced meal or snack that includes both protein and carbs.

3. Post-Exercise Nutrition: Consume a combination of carbohydrates and protein after workouts to replenish glycogen stores and promote muscle recovery.

4. Hydration: Stay hydrated before, during, and after exercise to support optimal performance and prevent dehydration.

Meal Planning Strategies for Active Individuals with Diabetes

Follow these meal planning strategies to optimize nutrition for exercise:

1. Pre-Exercise Meals and Snacks: Consume a carbohydrate-rich snack 30-60 minutes before exercise to fuel muscles. Examples include a banana, whole grain toast with peanut butter, or yogurt with berries.

2. Post-Exercise Recovery: Refuel with a balanced meal or snack within 30-60 minutes after exercise. Include carbohydrates (such as whole grains or fruits) and lean protein (such as chicken, fish, or tofu) to promote muscle recovery and glycogen replenishment.

3. Hydration: Drink water before, during, and after exercise to stay hydrated. Consider sports drinks if exercising intensely or for prolonged periods to replace electrolytes.

4. Balanced Meals and Snacks: Incorporate a mix of carbohydrates, protein, and healthy fats into meals and snacks to support sustained energy levels and blood sugar control throughout the day.

Sample Exercise-Focused Meal Plan for Diabetes

Here's an example of an exercise-focused meal plan for individuals with diabetes:

Breakfast:
- Oatmeal topped with sliced strawberries and almonds
- Scrambled eggs with spinach
- Herbal tea or black coffee

Mid-Morning Snack:
- Greek yogurt paired with a small amount of granola

Lunch:
- Grilled chicken salad with mixed greens, cherry tomatoes, cucumbers, and quinoa
- Olive oil and vinegar dressing
- Sparkling water with lemon or lime

Afternoon Snack:

- Whole grain crackers with hummus and sliced bell peppers

Dinner:
- Baked salmon with lemon and herbs
- Roasted Brussels sprouts and sweet potatoes
- Brown rice pilaf
- Sparkling water or herbal tea

Evening Snack:
- Apple slices with almond butter

Tips for Incorporating Exercise into Daily Routine

1. Choose Activities You Enjoy: Engage in activities you find enjoyable to stay motivated and committed to your exercise routine.
2. Set Realistic Goals: Start with manageable goals and gradually increase intensity, duration, and frequency over time.
3. Schedule Workouts: Block out time for exercise in your daily schedule to make it a priority.
4. Stay Consistent: Aim for regular, consistent exercise to maximize health benefits and blood sugar control.
5. Monitor Blood Sugar Levels: Check blood sugar levels before and after exercise to

understand how your body responds and make necessary adjustments to your meal plan and medication regimen.

Exercise is a vital component of diabetes management, synergizing with meal planning to optimize blood sugar control and overall health. By understanding the impact of exercise on meal planning and implementing practical strategies, individuals with diabetes can achieve better outcomes, improve quality of life, and reduce the risk of complications. Incorporating regular physical activity into a diabetes management routine empowers individuals to take control of their health and well-being, fostering a balanced and fulfilling lifestyle. With commitment, knowledge, and support, harnessing the power of exercise alongside meal planning becomes an integral part of thriving with diabetes.

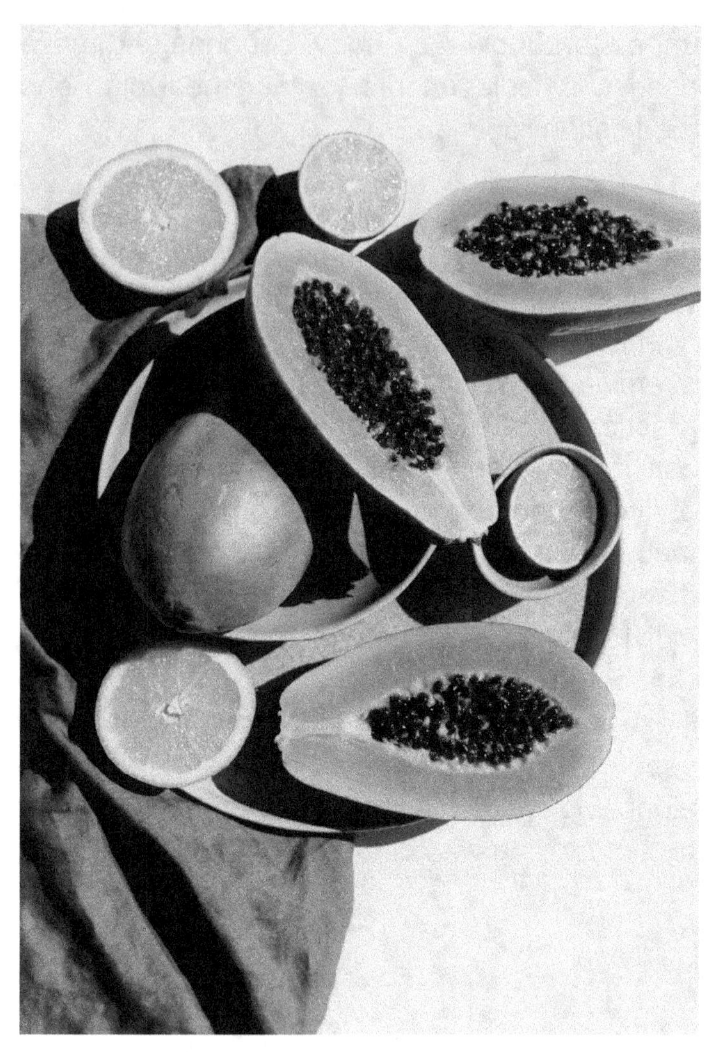

Chapter Ten

Mindful Eating and Emotional Well-being

For individuals who are newly diagnosed with diabetes, adopting mindful eating practices can be transformative in promoting emotional well-being and supporting overall health. Mindful eating involves paying attention to the present moment, savoring each bite, and cultivating a positive relationship with food. This comprehensive guide explores the intersection of mindful eating and emotional well-being within the context of a diabetes meal plan, offering practical insights, strategies, and meal ideas to empower individuals on their journey towards optimal health.

Understanding Mindful Eating

Mindful eating is rooted in the principles of mindfulness, emphasizing awareness and non-judgmental observation of thoughts, emotions, and sensations related to eating. Key aspects of mindful eating include:

1.   Present-Moment   Awareness: Bringing attention to the sensory experience of eating, including taste, texture, and aroma.
2. Non-Judgmental Observation: Cultivating a compassionate   and   non-critical   attitude towards food choices and eating behaviors.
3. Recognizing Hunger and Fullness Cues: Tuning into physical hunger and satiety signals to guide eating decisions.
4. Emotional Regulation: Developing healthier responses to emotional triggers and stressors through mindful eating practices.

The Connection Between Mindful Eating and Emotional Well-being

Emotional well-being is closely linked to how we nourish our bodies and relate to food. A healthy relationship with food is fostered via mindful eating, which can:

1. Reduce Emotional Eating: By increasing awareness of emotional triggers for eating, individuals can develop healthier coping mechanisms and reduce reliance on food for emotional comfort.
2. Enhance Satisfaction and Enjoyment: By savoring each bite and eating with awareness,

individuals derive greater satisfaction and pleasure from meals.

3. Improve Self-Regulation: Mindful eating promotes self-awareness and self-compassion, supporting healthier eating behaviors and emotional regulation.

4. Reduce Stress and Anxiety: Mindful eating practices can help manage stress and anxiety by promoting relaxation and reducing reactivity to emotional stimuli.

Practical Strategies for Mindful Eating

Incorporate these strategies into your diabetes meal plan to cultivate mindful eating habits:

1. Eat Without Distractions: Avoid eating in front of screens or while multitasking. Instead, focus on the sensory experience of eating.

2. Practice Portion Control: Use smaller plates and utensils to control portion sizes and prevent overeating.

3. Chew Slowly and Thoroughly: Take time to chew each bite thoroughly, allowing flavors to fully develop and promoting digestion.

4. Pause Between Bites: Put down utensils between bites and check in with hunger and fullness cues before continuing to eat.

5. Engage Your Senses: Notice colors, textures, and flavors of foods. To enjoy dining to the fullest, engage all of your senses.
6. Mindful Grocery Shopping: Plan meals ahead, make a shopping list, and shop for nutritious ingredients mindfully.
7. Cook with Intention: Prepare meals with care and attention, focusing on nourishing your body and enjoying the process of cooking.

Meal Planning with Mindful Eating Principles

Integrate mindful eating principles into your diabetes meal plan with these meal ideas:

Breakfast:
- Greek yogurt parfait with layers of fresh berries, nuts, and a drizzle of honey
- Herbal tea or black coffee

Mid-Morning Snack:
- An apple sliced and topped with almond butter.

Lunch:
- Quinoa salad with roasted vegetables (bell peppers, zucchini, and cherry tomatoes) and grilled chicken

- Balsamic vinaigrette dressing
- Sparkling water with lemon or lime

Afternoon Snack:
- Raw vegetable sticks (carrots, celery, and cucumber) with hummus

Dinner:
- Baked salmon with a lemon-dill sauce
- Steamed broccoli and cauliflower
- Whole grain couscous
- Sparkling water or herbal tea

Evening Snack:
- Dark chocolate square with a handful of mixed nuts

Tips for Enhancing Emotional Well-being Through Mindful Eating

1. Practice Gratitude: Express gratitude for the nourishing qualities of food and the act of eating.
2. Release Judgment: Approach eating with curiosity and openness, letting go of self-criticism and judgment.
3. Listen to Your Body: Tune into hunger and fullness cues, eating when hungry and stopping when satisfied.

4. Cultivate Self-Compassion: Be kind to yourself and acknowledge that eating is a natural and essential part of self-care.
5. Mindful Breathing: Practice deep breathing exercises before meals to calm the mind and body.
6. Seek Support: Connect with a registered dietitian or counselor specializing in mindful eating for additional guidance and support.

Incorporating Mindful Eating into Everyday Life

Make mindful eating a part of your daily routine by incorporating these practices:

1. Set Intentions: Begin meals with a moment of reflection or intention-setting to cultivate mindfulness.
2. Create Rituals: Establish mealtime rituals, such as setting the table mindfully or lighting a candle before eating.
3. Practice Gratitude: Take a moment to express gratitude for the food you are about to eat and the nourishment it provides.
4. Eat Mindfully: Slow down and savor each bite, noticing flavors, textures, and sensations.

5. Reflect: After eating, reflect on how you feel physically and emotionally, without judgment or criticism.

Mindful eating is a powerful tool for enhancing emotional well-being and supporting diabetes management. By incorporating mindful eating practices into your diabetes meal plan, you can develop a healthier relationship with food, reduce emotional eating, and cultivate greater satisfaction and enjoyment from meals. Embrace mindfulness as a holistic approach to diabetes care, integrating awareness, compassion, and intention into your eating habits. With dedication and practice, mindful eating can transform mealtime into a nourishing and fulfilling experience that promotes overall health and emotional well-being for individuals living with diabetes.

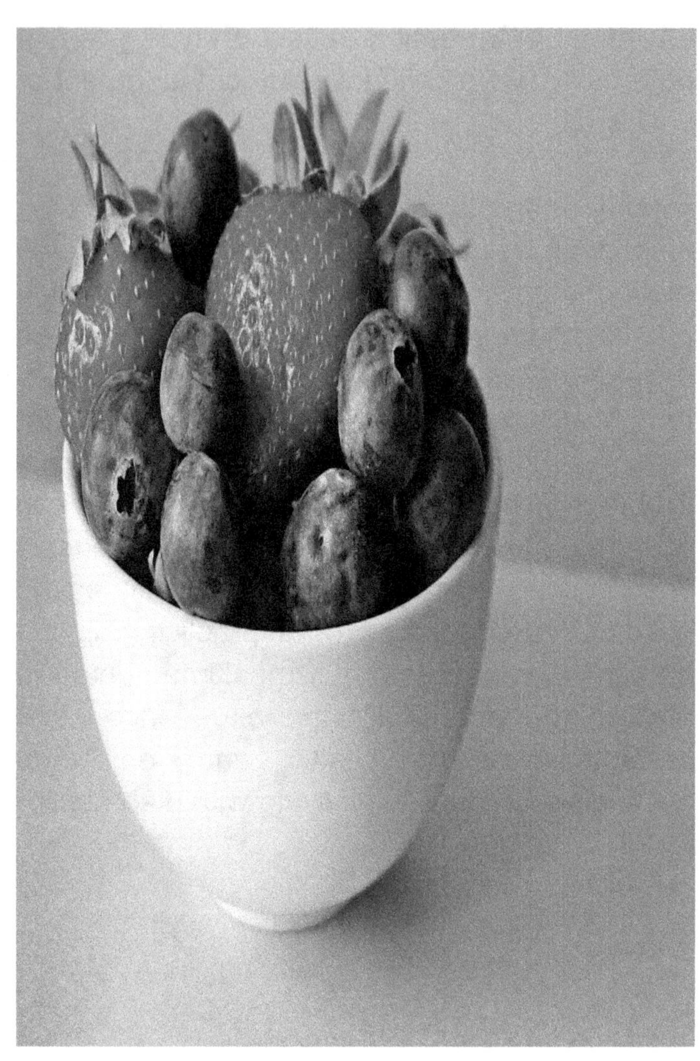

Chapter Eleven

Healthy Cooking Techniques

Cooking plays a pivotal role in managing diabetes, allowing individuals to create delicious and balanced meals that support blood sugar control and overall health. Adopting healthy cooking techniques can transform everyday ingredients into nourishing dishes without compromising flavor. In this comprehensive guide, we will explore a variety of healthy cooking techniques tailored for individuals who are newly diagnosed with diabetes, providing practical insights, tips, and recipes to inspire culinary creativity and promote well-being.

Importance of Healthy Cooking for Diabetes Management

Cooking at home using healthy techniques offers numerous benefits for individuals with diabetes:

1. Control Over Ingredients: Cooking at home allows individuals to control the quality and quantity of ingredients, reducing the intake of unhealthy fats, sodium, and added sugars.

2. Nutrient Retention: Healthy cooking techniques preserve the nutritional value of foods, maximizing the availability of essential vitamins, minerals, and antioxidants.

3. Enhanced Flavor: By using wholesome ingredients and flavorful seasonings, home-cooked meals can be as delicious as they are nutritious, making healthy eating enjoyable and sustainable.

4. Promotes Portion Control: Cooking at home encourages portion control, preventing overeating and supporting weight management.

Essential Healthy Cooking Techniques for Diabetes

Incorporate these healthy cooking techniques into your diabetes meal plan to create balanced and satisfying meals:

1. Grilling: Grilling imparts a smoky flavor to foods without adding extra fats. Use lean proteins like chicken breast, fish, or vegetables marinated in herbs and spices.

2. Roasting: Roasting vegetables and proteins intensifies their flavors. Toss vegetables like

broccoli, cauliflower, or Brussels sprouts with olive oil and roast until tender and caramelized.

3. Steaming: Steaming preserves the natural color, texture, and nutrients of vegetables. Steam broccoli, carrots, or spinach until just tender, and season with lemon juice and herbs.

4. Sautéing: Use minimal oil or cooking spray to sauté vegetables and proteins. Start with aromatics like garlic and onions, then add vegetables like bell peppers, zucchini, or mushrooms.

5. Baking: Baking is a healthy cooking method that requires little added fat. Bake whole grains like quinoa or brown rice, or prepare baked fish with a crust of herbs and whole-wheat breadcrumbs.

6. Stir-Frying: Stir-frying uses high heat and minimal oil to cook vegetables and proteins quickly. Use a mix of colorful vegetables and lean proteins like tofu or shrimp, seasoned with ginger and soy sauce.

7. Poaching: Poaching involves cooking foods in simmering liquid, such as water or broth.

Poach chicken breasts or fish fillets with herbs and spices for a tender and flavorful dish.

8. Broiling: Broiling uses intense heat from above to cook foods quickly. Broil salmon fillets or chicken breast until golden and cooked through, adding a squeeze of lemon juice for freshness.

Tips for Healthy Cooking with Diabetes

Follow these practical tips to make healthy cooking enjoyable and accessible:

1. Use Healthy Fats: Opt for heart-healthy fats like olive oil, avocado oil, or canola oil instead of butter or lard.
2. Choose Lean Proteins: Select lean proteins such as skinless poultry, fish, tofu, or legumes to reduce saturated fat intake.
3. Incorporate Whole Grains: Replace refined grains with whole grains like quinoa, brown rice, or whole wheat pasta for added fiber and nutrients.
4. Season with Herbs and Spices: Flavor foods with herbs, spices, and citrus instead of salt or sugar to enhance taste without excess sodium.
5. Limit Added Sugars: Use natural sweeteners like stevia, monk fruit, or small amounts of

honey or maple syrup instead of refined sugars.

6. Experiment with Plant-Based Meals: Explore plant-based cooking with meals centered around vegetables, legumes, and whole grains for variety and nutrient density.

7. Practice Portion Control: Use smaller plates and measure portions to prevent overeating and support blood sugar control.

Sample Recipes for Healthy Cooking with Diabetes

Try these diabetes-friendly recipes showcasing healthy cooking techniques:

Grilled Lemon Herb Chicken:
- Marinate chicken breasts in a mixture of lemon juice, garlic, and fresh herbs.
- Grill until cooked through and serve with steamed green beans and quinoa pilaf.

Roasted Vegetable Medley:
- Toss cauliflower florets, bell peppers, and cherry tomatoes with olive oil, garlic, and Italian herbs.
- Roast in the oven until caramelized and serve as a colorful side dish.

Stir-Fried Tofu and Vegetable Stir-Fry:
- Sauté tofu cubes with broccoli, snap peas, and bell peppers in a sesame-ginger sauce.
- For a filling supper, serve over brown rice or cauliflower rice.

Baked Salmon with Dill and Lemon:
- Place salmon fillets on a baking sheet and season with fresh dill, lemon zest, and a drizzle of olive oil.
- Bake until flaky and serve with a side of steamed asparagus.

Healthy cooking techniques are essential tools for individuals managing diabetes, offering a pathway to flavorful and nutrient-dense meals that support blood sugar control and overall well-being. By incorporating grilling, roasting, steaming, and other healthy cooking methods into your diabetes meal plan, you can create delicious dishes that nourish the body and delight the taste buds. Embrace the joy of cooking with wholesome ingredients, vibrant flavors, and mindful preparation to cultivate a positive relationship with food and promote optimal health. With creativity, knowledge, and a passion for nutritious eating, healthy cooking becomes a cornerstone of diabetes management and a source of culinary inspiration for a lifetime.

Chapter Twelve

Meal Planning for Weight Management

Effective meal planning plays a vital role in managing weight while living with diabetes. For individuals who are newly diagnosed, understanding how to create a balanced meal plan that supports weight management and blood sugar control is essential for overall health and well-being. This comprehensive guide explores the principles of meal planning for weight management within the context of diabetes, providing practical strategies, tips, and meal ideas to empower individuals on their journey towards a healthier lifestyle.

Importance of Meal Planning for Weight Management with Diabetes

Managing weight is particularly important for individuals with diabetes, as excess body weight can contribute to insulin resistance and increase the risk of complications. Meal planning for weight management offers several benefits:

1. Controlled Caloric Intake: Meal planning allows for portion control and mindful eating, which can help regulate calorie intake and support weight loss or maintenance.

2. Balanced Nutrient Intake: A well-planned meal helps ensure that individuals receive essential nutrients while avoiding excessive calories, fats, or sugars.

3. Stabilized Blood Sugar Levels: Choosing the right foods in appropriate portions helps prevent blood sugar spikes and crashes, promoting stable energy levels and insulin sensitivity.

4. Sustained Energy: A balanced meal plan supports sustained energy throughout the day, reducing cravings and overeating.

Principles of Meal Planning for Weight Management

Follow these principles to create a diabetes meal plan that supports weight management:

1. Balanced Macronutrients: Include a balance of carbohydrates, proteins, and healthy fats in each meal to support satiety and prevent blood sugar fluctuations.

2. Portion Control: Be mindful of portion sizes and calorie intake, especially for high-calorie foods like fats and carbohydrates.

3. Emphasize Whole Foods: Choose whole, minimally processed foods such as fruits, vegetables, whole grains, lean proteins, and healthy fats.

4. Fiber-Rich Foods: Incorporate fiber-rich foods like vegetables, fruits, whole grains, and legumes to promote fullness and digestive health.

5. Limit Added Sugars and Saturated Fats: Minimize consumption of foods high in added sugars, unhealthy fats, and refined carbohydrates.

6. Regular Meals and Snacks: Eat at regular intervals throughout the day to prevent excessive hunger and overeating.

Strategies for Meal Planning for Weight Management

Use these strategies to create a diabetes meal plan that supports weight management:

1. Plan Ahead: Schedule some time each week to organize your snacks and meals. Use a meal planning template to organize your menu and grocery list.

2. Include Variety: Incorporate a variety of foods from different food groups to ensure balanced nutrition and prevent boredom.

3. Choose Low-Glycemic Index (GI) Foods: Opt for low-GI foods like whole grains, legumes, non-starchy vegetables, and fruits to help control blood sugar levels and promote satiety.

4. Control Portions: Use measuring cups, spoons, or visual cues (like the palm of your hand) to control portion sizes and avoid overeating.

5. Stay Hydrated: Drink plenty of water throughout the day to stay hydrated and support metabolism.

6. Be Mindful of Snacks: Choose healthy snacks that are nutrient-dense and portion-controlled to curb cravings between meals.

Sample Meal Plan for Weight Management with Diabetes

Here's an example of a diabetes-friendly meal plan focused on weight management:

Breakfast:
- Spinach and feta omelet made with egg whites
- Whole grain toast with avocado spread
- Sliced tomatoes and cucumbers
- Herbal tea or black coffee

Mid-Morning Snack:
- Greek yogurt with mixed berries
Lunch:
- Mixed greens, cucumbers, cherry tomatoes, and grilled chicken salad with a light vinaigrette dressing.
- Quinoa pilaf
- Sparkling water with lemon or lime
Afternoon Snack:
- Hummus with carrot and celery sticks

Dinner:
- Baked salmon with lemon and herbs
- Steamed broccoli and cauliflower
- Brown rice or cauliflower rice
- Sparkling water or herbal tea

Evening Snack:
- Sliced apple with almond butter

Tips for Successful Weight Management with Diabetes
1. Monitor Portion Sizes: Use smaller plates and bowls to control portion sizes and prevent overeating.
2. Eat Mindfully: Slow down and savor each bite, paying attention to hunger and fullness cues.

3. Stay Active: Incorporate regular physical activity into your routine to support weight management and overall health.

4. Limit Liquid Calories: Avoid sugary drinks and alcoholic beverages, opting for water, herbal tea, or sparkling water instead.

5. Seek Support: Consult with a registered dietitian or healthcare provider for personalized guidance and support in managing weight with diabetes.

Meal planning is a powerful tool for managing weight and promoting overall health for individuals living with diabetes. By incorporating balanced meals, portion control, and healthy eating strategies into your daily routine, you can achieve weight management goals while supporting blood sugar control and reducing the risk of complications. Embrace the principles of mindful eating, variety, and moderation to create a sustainable diabetes meal plan that nourishes the body and promotes well-being. With dedication, knowledge, and support, meal planning becomes an empowering aspect of diabetes management and a pathway to a healthier, more fulfilling life.

Chapter Thirteen

Family and Social Support

Being newly diagnosed with diabetes can be overwhelming, but having strong family and social support can make a significant difference in navigating this journey. Family and friends play a crucial role in providing emotional encouragement, practical assistance, and motivation for individuals managing diabetes. In this comprehensive guide, we will explore the importance of family and social support in diabetes management, offering practical tips, insights, and strategies to foster a supportive environment for individuals newly diagnosed with diabetes.

The Importance of Family and Social Support

Family and social support are instrumental in diabetes management for several reasons:

1. Emotional Well-being: Supportive relationships can alleviate stress, anxiety, and depression associated with diabetes diagnosis and management.

2. Practical Assistance: Family members can assist with meal preparation, grocery shopping, medication reminders, and doctor's appointments.

3. Encouragement for Lifestyle Changes: Positive reinforcement and motivation from loved ones can facilitate adherence to healthy eating, exercise, and medication regimens.

4. Role Modeling: Family members who model healthy behaviors can inspire positive lifestyle changes in individuals with diabetes.

5. Social Connection: Engaging with supportive social networks can reduce feelings of isolation and promote a sense of belonging.

Ways Family and Social Support Contribute to Diabetes Management

1. Emotional Support:

- Listening without judgment and offering empathy and understanding.

- Offering consolation and support when things are hard.

- Participating in open and honest conversations about feelings and concerns related to diabetes.

2. Practical Support:

- Assisting with meal planning and preparation of diabetes-friendly meals.

- Accompanying to medical appointments and helping manage medications.

- Joining in physical activities such as walks, bike rides, or exercise classes.

3. Educational Support:

- Learning about diabetes together as a family to better understand the condition and treatment.

- Sharing resources, articles, and books about diabetes and healthy living.

4. Role Modeling Healthy Behaviors:

- Adopting healthy eating habits and encouraging balanced meals for the entire family.

- Engaging in regular physical activity as a family to promote an active lifestyle.

Strategies for Building Family and Social Support

1. Open Communication:

- Foster open communication about diabetes-related concerns, challenges, and goals within the family.

- Encourage asking questions and seeking clarification about diabetes management.

2. Education and Awareness:
   - Educate family members and close friends about diabetes, its management, and the importance of support.
   - Share information about healthy eating, physical activity, and blood sugar monitoring.

3. Involvement in Meal Planning:
   - Involve family members in meal planning and preparation to ensure diabetes-friendly and enjoyable meals for everyone.
   - Experiment with new recipes and cooking techniques together.

4. Physical Activity as a Family:
   - Plan regular family activities that promote physical activity, such as hiking, swimming, or playing sports.
   - Make physical activity enjoyable and inclusive for all family members.

5. Celebrating Achievements:
   - Acknowledge and celebrate milestones and achievements in diabetes management.
   - Recognize efforts made towards healthier lifestyle choices.

Tips for Encouraging Social Support

1. Join Diabetes Support Groups:
   - Encourage participation in local or online diabetes support groups to connect with others facing similar challenges.

2. Educate Close Friends and Colleagues:
   - Share information about diabetes with close friends, colleagues, and peers to raise awareness and foster understanding.

3. Seek Professional Counseling:
   - Consider family counseling or therapy sessions to address emotional challenges and strengthen relationships.

4. Set Boundaries:
   - Communicate clear boundaries and preferences regarding diabetes management with family and friends.

Navigating Social Events and Gatherings

1. Communicate Dietary Needs:
   - Inform hosts or event organizers about dietary restrictions and preferences related to diabetes.

2. Plan Ahead:

 - Bring diabetes-friendly dishes or snacks to social gatherings to ensure healthy options are available.

3. Manage Stress:

 - Practice stress-reducing techniques such as deep breathing, meditation, or mindfulness during social events.

Family and social support are invaluable resources for individuals newly diagnosed with diabetes, providing emotional encouragement, practical assistance, and motivation for effective diabetes management. By fostering open communication, educating loved ones, and involving them in diabetes-related activities, individuals can build a strong support network that promotes overall well-being and enhances quality of life. Embrace the power of family and social support in your diabetes journey, and remember that you are not alone. Together, we can navigate the challenges of diabetes and celebrate the successes that come with a supportive and understanding community.

Chapter Fourteen

Tracking Progress and Adjusting Meal Plans

Tracking progress and making necessary adjustments to meal plans are essential components of effective diabetes management, especially for individuals who are newly diagnosed. Monitoring key indicators such as blood sugar levels, weight, and overall health outcomes allows for personalized adjustments that optimize blood sugar control and promote overall well-being. In this comprehensive guide, we will explore the importance of tracking progress and adjusting meal plans in diabetes management, providing practical insights, strategies, and tips to empower individuals on their journey towards health and vitality.

Importance of Tracking Progress in Diabetes Management

Tracking progress is critical for several reasons:

1. Assessment of Blood Sugar Levels: Regular monitoring of blood glucose levels provides insights into how different foods and lifestyle factors impact blood sugar control.

2. Evaluation of Weight Changes: Tracking weight fluctuations helps determine the effectiveness of dietary modifications and lifestyle interventions on weight management.

3. Identification of Trends and Patterns: Monitoring trends over time helps identify patterns related to meal timing, portion sizes, and carbohydrate intake.

4. Early Detection of Complications: Tracking progress allows for early detection of potential complications such as hyperglycemia or hypoglycemia, enabling timely adjustments to meal plans and treatment regimens.

5. Personalized Diabetes Management: By tracking progress, individuals can tailor their meal plans and lifestyle choices to meet specific health goals and preferences.

Tools for Tracking Progress:

Utilize the following tools and techniques to monitor progress effectively:

1. Blood Glucose Monitoring Devices: Use glucometers to measure blood sugar levels

before and after meals, as well as at different times throughout the day.

2. Food and Blood Sugar Journals: Keep a detailed record of meals, snacks, portion sizes, and corresponding blood sugar readings to identify trends and patterns.

3. Weight Tracking: Use a scale to monitor weight changes over time and assess the impact of dietary modifications on weight management.

4. Physical Activity Logs: Maintain a log of daily physical activity, including type, duration, and intensity, to evaluate its influence on blood sugar levels and overall health.

Strategies for Adjusting Meal Plans

Make informed adjustments to meal plans based on tracked progress and health outcomes:

1. Consult with Healthcare Providers: Collaborate with registered dietitians, endocrinologists, or diabetes educators to interpret progress data and make appropriate adjustments.

2. Review Blood Sugar Readings: Analyze blood glucose readings to identify postprandial spikes or patterns of hypoglycemia and modify meal composition accordingly.

3. Assess Weight Changes: Evaluate weight fluctuations and adjust portion sizes or calorie intake to support weight management goals.

4. Modify Carbohydrate Intake: Fine-tune carbohydrate consumption based on blood sugar responses and physical activity levels to optimize glycemic control.

5. Experiment with Meal Timing: Adjust meal timing and frequency to prevent blood sugar fluctuations and promote sustained energy levels throughout the day.

6. Incorporate Personal Preferences: Consider individual food preferences, cultural influences, and lifestyle factors when making meal plan adjustments to ensure adherence and satisfaction.

Tips for Effective Progress Tracking and Adjustment:

1. Consistency is Key: Maintain a consistent tracking routine to capture meaningful data over time and identify long-term trends.

2. Set Realistic Goals: Establish achievable goals based on tracked progress and adjust meal plans gradually to promote sustainable changes.

3. Educate and Empower: Educate yourself and loved ones about the importance of

progress tracking and involve them in the adjustment process for added support.

4. Celebrate Milestones: Celebrate achievements and milestones along the diabetes management journey to stay motivated and inspired.

5. Stay Flexible: Be open to experimentation and adaptability when making adjustments to meal plans to find what works best for individual needs and preferences.

Sample Meal Plan Adjustment Strategies:
Consider the following sample strategies for adjusting meal plans based on tracked progress:

1. Reducing Portion Sizes: Decrease portion sizes of high-carbohydrate foods to manage blood sugar levels and support weight loss goals.

2. Substituting Ingredients: Replace refined carbohydrates with whole grains or fiber-rich alternatives to improve glycemic control and promote satiety.

3. Balancing Macronutrients: Adjust the ratio of carbohydrates, proteins, and fats in meals to achieve optimal blood sugar regulation and sustained energy.

4. Experimenting with Meal Timing: Incorporate smaller, more frequent meals or snacks to prevent blood sugar fluctuations and support metabolism.
5. Monitoring Hydration: Stay hydrated and avoid sugary beverages to maintain optimal blood sugar levels and overall health.

Tracking progress and making informed adjustments to meal plans are integral components of effective diabetes management, empowering individuals to optimize blood sugar control, promote weight management, and enhance overall well-being. By utilizing tools for progress tracking, collaborating with healthcare providers, and implementing personalized adjustment strategies, individuals can tailor their meal plans to meet specific health goals and preferences. Embrace the dynamic nature of diabetes management, and remember that progress tracking is not only about monitoring numbers but also about fostering a deeper understanding of individual responses to dietary choices and lifestyle modifications. With dedication, knowledge, and support, individuals can achieve lasting success in diabetes management through proactive progress tracking and thoughtful meal plan adjustments.

Conclusion

"The Diabetes Meal Plan for the Newly Diagnosed" offers a comprehensive and invaluable resource for individuals embarking on their journey of managing diabetes. Throughout this book, we have explored a wide range of topics essential to understanding, planning, and executing a diabetes-friendly meal plan that not only supports optimal blood sugar control but also promotes overall health and well-being.

From understanding diabetes and its impact on the body to delving into the intricacies of mindful eating, healthy cooking techniques, and meal planning strategies, this book has provided practical insights, tips, and delicious recipes tailored specifically for those navigating the challenges of a new diabetes diagnosis.

We have emphasized the importance of family and social support in diabetes management, recognizing the pivotal role that loved ones play in providing emotional encouragement, practical assistance, and motivation. Engaging with a supportive network can make a significant difference in successfully managing diabetes and achieving health goals.

Tracking progress and adjusting meal plans based on individual needs and responses have been highlighted as critical components of effective diabetes management. By utilizing tools for progress tracking, consulting healthcare providers, and implementing personalized adjustment strategies, individuals can tailor their meal plans to optimize blood sugar control and overall health outcomes.

Ultimately, managing diabetes is a journey that requires dedication, knowledge, and ongoing support. With the right information, resources, and a proactive approach to meal planning and lifestyle modifications, individuals can take charge of their health and embrace a fulfilling life with diabetes.

This book serves as a guide and companion for individuals newly diagnosed with diabetes, offering empowerment, inspiration, and practical solutions to navigate the challenges and embrace the opportunities of diabetes management. By implementing the principles and strategies outlined in this book, readers can embark on a path towards improved health, well-being, and a thriving life with diabetes. Remember, each step taken towards healthier choices and mindful living is a step towards a brighter and healthier future.